HOME WORKOUT FOR BEGINNERS:
The Ultimate Workout Guide For Beginners
At home.

Chapman Parker

Table of contents

Chapter 1

WHY IS EXERCISE IMPORTANT

Here are the top 10 ways regular exercise helps your body and brain.

1. Exercise may make you feel happy
Exercise has been proved to boost your mood and minimize emotions of despair, anxiety, and stress

It creates changes in the areas of the brain that control stress and anxiety. It may also enhance brain sensitivity to the neurotransmitters serotonin and norepinephrine, which decrease symptoms of despair.

Additionally, exercise may enhance the synthesis of endorphins, which are known to help promote happy moods and lower the perception of pain.

Interestingly, it doesn't matter how tough your exercise is. It appears that exercise may enhance your mood no matter the intensity of physical activity.

In fact, in research on 24 women diagnosed with depression, the exercise of any intensity dramatically improved symptoms of sadness.

The effects of exercise on mood are so potent that choosing to exercise (or not) even makes a difference over short periods.

One assessment of 19 research indicated that active adults who quit exercising regularly reported substantial increases in symptoms of despair and anxiety, even after just a few weeks.

SUMMARY\sExercising frequently may enhance your mood and lessen symptoms of anxiety and despair.

2. Exercise may assist with weight reduction
Some studies have indicated that inactivity is a key contributor to weight gain and obesity.

To comprehend the influence of exercise on weight loss, it is vital to understand the link between activity and energy expenditure (spending) (spending).

Your body spends energy in three ways:

Digesting food.
Exercising.
Maintaining biological functions, such as your pulse, and breathing.

While dieting, a decreased calorie intake can lower your metabolic rate, which might temporarily postpone weight reduction. On the contrary, regular exercise has been demonstrated to raise your metabolic rate, which may burn more calories to help you lose weight.

Additionally, studies have shown that combining aerobic exercise with strength training may enhance fat reduction and muscle mass maintenance, which is vital for keeping the weight off and retaining lean muscle composition.

SUMMARY\sExercise is vital to sustaining a healthy metabolism and burning more calories each day. It also helps you maintain your muscle mass and weight reduction.

3. Exercise is healthy for your muscles and bones:\sExercise has a critical function in creating and maintaining strong muscles and bones.

Activities like weightlifting may boost muscle development when accompanied by proper protein intake.

This is because exercise helps release hormones that enhance your muscles' capacity to absorb amino acids. This helps them flourish and inhibits their breakdown.

As individuals age, they tend to lose muscle mass and function, which may contribute to an increased risk of injury. Practicing regular physical exercise is vital to decreasing muscle loss and preserving strength as you age.

Exercise also helps improve bone density while you're younger, in addition to helping prevent osteoporosis later in life.

Some studies show that high-impact exercise (such as gymnastics or running) or odd-impact sports (such as soccer and basketball) may assist produce a greater bone density than no-impact sports like swimming and cycling.

SUMMARY

Physical exercise helps you create muscles and healthy bones. It may also help prevent osteoporosis.

4. Exercise may raise your energy levels:\sExercise can be a significant energy booster for many individuals, even those with different medical issues.

One earlier research indicated that 6 weeks of regular exercise improved symptoms of exhaustion for 36 persons who previously experienced continuous weariness.

And let's not forget the amazing heart and lung health advantages of exercise. Aerobic exercise enhances the cardiovascular system and promotes lung function, which may greatly aid energy levels.

As you move more, your heart pumps more blood, supplying more oxygen to your working muscles. With regular exercise, your heart becomes more efficient and adept at moving oxygen into your blood, making your muscles more efficient.

Over time, this aerobic training results in less demand on your lungs, and it requires less energy to perform the same activities — one of the reasons you're less likely to get short of breath during vigorous activity.

Additionally, exercise has been demonstrated to enhance energy levels in persons with various diseases, such as cancer.

SUMMARY
Engaging in regular physical exercise might enhance your energy levels.

5. Exercise may lessen your risk of chronic illness:\sLack of regular physical exercise is the main cause of chronic disease.

Regular exercise has been demonstrated to enhance insulin sensitivity, heart health, and body composition. It may help lower blood pressure and cholesterol levels.

More precisely, exercise may help lessen or avoid the following chronic health issues.

Type 2 diabetes.
Regular aerobic exercise may postpone or prevent type 2 diabetes. It also provides great health advantages for those with type 1 diabetes. Resistance training for type 2 diabetes involves improvements in fat mass, blood pressure, lean body mass, insulin resistance, and glycemic management.
Heart illness.

Exercise decreases cardiovascular risk factors and is also a therapeutic therapy for persons with cardiovascular disease.
Many forms of cancer.
Exercise may help lower the risk of numerous cancers, including breast,

colorectal, endometrial, gallbladder, kidney, lung, liver, ovarian, pancreatic, prostate, thyroid, gastric, and esophageal cancer.
High cholesterol.
Regular moderate intensity physical exercise may enhance HDL (good) cholesterol while preserving or balancing increases in LDL (bad) cholesterol. Research supports the hypothesis that high-intensity aerobic exercise is required to reduce LDL levels.

Hypertension: \sParticipating in regular aerobic exercise may reduce resting systolic BP 5–7 mmHg among patients with hypertension.
In contrast, a lack of regular exercise even in the short term may lead to considerable increases in belly fat, which may raise the risk of type 2 diabetes and heart disease.

That's why regular physical exercise is suggested to reduce abdominal fat and lessen the chance of getting these diseases.

SUMMARY\sDaily physical exercise is vital to maintaining a healthy weight and minimizing the risk of chronic illness.

6. Exercise may assist skin health:\sYour skin can be influenced by the amount of oxidative stress in your body.

Oxidative stress arises when the body's antioxidant defenses cannot fully repair the cell damage produced by chemicals known as free radicals. This might harm the structure of the cells and badly influence your skin.

Even though extreme and strenuous physical activity might add to oxidative damage, frequent moderate exercise can improve your body's production of natural antioxidants, which assist protect cells.

In the same manner, exercise may promote blood flow and generate skin cell changes that can help postpone the appearance of skin aging.

SUMMARY\sModerate exercise may give antioxidant protection and stimulate blood flow, which helps preserve your skin and prevent indications of aging.

7. Exercise may enhance your brain health and memory: Exercise can increase brain function and safeguard memory and cognitive abilities.

To begin with, it boosts your heart rate, which enhances the flow of blood and oxygen to your brain. It may also boost the synthesis of hormones that enhance the proliferation of brain cells.

Plus, the capacity of exercise to avoid chronic illness might translate into advantages for your brain, as its function can be impaired by these disorders.

Regular physical exercise is particularly crucial in older persons as aging — along with oxidative stress and inflammation — causes changes in brain structure and function.

Exercise has been proven to encourage the hippocampus, a portion of the brain that's crucial for memory and learning, to increase in size, which may aid enhance mental performance in older individuals.

Lastly, exercise has been proven to minimize changes in the brain that may lead to illnesses like Alzheimer's disease and dementia.

SUMMARY
Regular exercise boosts blood flow to the brain and enhances brain health and memory. Among elderly persons, it may help preserve mental function.

8. Exercise can help with relaxation and sleep quality: Regular exercise can help you relax and sleep better.

Concerning sleep quality, the energy depletion (loss) that happens during exercise drives restorative processes during sleep.

Moreover, the rise in body temperature that happens during exercise is suggested to enhance sleep quality by helping body temperature decline during sleep

Much research on the effects of exercise on sleep has found similar findings.

One evaluation of six research revealed that engaging in an exercise training program helped enhance self-reported sleep quality and lowered sleep latency, which is the amount of time it takes to fall asleep.

One research done over 4 months indicated that both stretching and resistance exercise contributed to improvements in sleep for persons with chronic insomnia.

Getting back to sleep after awakening, sleep length, and sleep quality increased following both stretching and resistance exercises. Anxiety was also lowered in the stretching group.

What's more, partaking in regular exercise tends to help older folks, who are commonly impacted by sleep difficulties.

You may be versatile with the sort of workout you pick. It seems that either aerobic exercise alone or aerobic exercise mixed with strength training may both enhance sleep quality.

SUMMARY
Regular physical exercise, regardless of whether it is aerobic or a mix of aerobic and

resistance training, may help you sleep better and feel more invigorated throughout the day.

9. Exercise may lessen pain:\sAlthough chronic pain can be awful, exercise can help alleviate it.

In fact, for many years, the suggestion for managing chronic pain was rest and inactivity. However, new research demonstrates that exercise can reduce chronic pain.
One analysis of multiple research indicated that exercise may assist patients with chronic pain lessen their discomfort and enhance their quality of life.

Several studies also demonstrate that exercise may help reduce pain linked with different health issues, including chronic low back pain, fibromyalgia, and chronic soft tissue shoulder dysfunction, to mention a few.

Additionally, physical exercise may help enhance pain tolerance and reduce pain perception.

SUMMARY
Exercise has good benefits on the pain linked with numerous diseases. It may also boost pain tolerance.

10. Exercise helps foster a healthier sex life:\sExercise has been proved to improve sex desire.

Engaging in regular exercise helps strengthen the heart, increase blood circulation, tone muscles, and boost flexibility, all of which can improve your sex life.

Physical exercise may also increase sexual performance and sexual enjoyment while increasing the frequency of sexual activity.

Interestingly enough, one research revealed that regular exercise was connected with enhanced sexual function and desire in 405 postmenopausal women.

A study of 10 research also revealed that exercising for at least 160 minutes per week over 6 months might help considerably enhance erectile function in males.

What's more, another research revealed that a modest practice of a 6-minute walk around the home helped 41 men lessen their erectile dysfunction symptoms by 71%.

Yet another research revealed that women with polycystic ovarian syndrome, which may impair sex desire, improved their sex drive with regular strength exercise for 16 weeks.

SUMMARY\sExercise may assist increase sexual desire, function, and performance in men and women. It may also help lessen the risk of erectile dysfunction in males.

The bottom line
Exercise has great advantages that may enhance practically every area of your health. Regular physical exercise might improve the synthesis of hormones that make you feel happy and help you sleep better.

It may also:

boost your skin's look
help you lose weight and keep it off\sreduce the risk of chronic illness
enhance your sex life
And it doesn't take much activity to make a major effect on your health.

If you aim for 150 to 300 minutes of moderate-intensity aerobic exercise each week or 75 minutes of strenuous physical activity dispersed throughout the week, you'll fulfill the Department of Health and Human Services' activity recommendations for adults.

Moderate intensity aerobic exercise is anything that makes your heart pounding quicker, including walking, cycling, or swimming. Activities like jogging or engaging in a tough exercise class qualify for severe intensity.

Throw in at least 2 days of muscle-strengthening workouts encompassing all main muscle groups (legs, hips, back abdomen, chest, shoulders, and arms), and you'll surpass the standards.

You may use weights, resistance bands, or your bodyweight to execute muscle-strengthening exercises. These include squats, push-ups, shoulder presses, chest, presses, and planks.

Chapter 2

Plan making

4 basic steps to get started
You're just five steps away from a healthy
living.

You may start a fitness program as a novice
in simply five steps.

1. Assess your fitness level
You probably have some concept of how fit
you are. But testing and documenting
baseline fitness scores may provide you
standards against which to gauge your
development. To test your aerobic and

muscular fitness, flexibility, and body composition, try recording:

Your pulse rate before and soon after walking 1 mile (1.6 kilometers) (1.6 kilometers).
How long it takes to walk 1 mile, or how long it takes to run 1.5 miles (2.41 kilometers) (2.41 kilometers).

How many normal or modified pushups you can perform at a time?
How far you can stretch forward when sitting on the floor with your legs in front of you?
Your waist circumference, right above your hipbones.

2. Design your fitness regimen
It's simple to state that you'll work out every day. But you'll need a plan. As you develop your training routine, keep these principles in mind:

Consider your fitness objectives. Are you beginning a workout program to help reduce weight? Or do you have another motivation? Having defined objectives might help you assess your progress and remain motivated.

Create a balanced regimen. Get at least 150 minutes of moderate aerobic exercise or 75 minutes of intense aerobic activity a week, or a mix of moderate and strenuous activity. The rules recommended that you stretch out this activity over a week. To give even greater health benefits and to aid with weight reduction or sustaining weight loss, at least 300 minutes a week is advised.

But even tiny quantities of physical exercise are useful. Being active for little amounts of time throughout the day might build up to bring health benefits.

Start low and progress steadily. If you're just starting to exercise, start gently and advance steadily. If you have an injury or a medical condition, visit your doctor or an exercise therapist for assistance in devising a fitness program that progressively increases your range of motion, strength, and endurance.

Build movement into your everyday routine. Finding time to work out might be a problem. To make it easy, plan time to exercise like you would any other appointment. Plan to watch your favorite program.

Plan to incorporate varied activities. Different activities (cross-training) help keep exercise monotony at bay. Cross-training employs low-impact kinds of activities. Plan to alternate among activities that focus on various portions of your body.

Allow time for healing. Many individuals start exercising with feverish fervor — working out too long or too intensively — then quit when their muscles and joints get uncomfortable or damaged. Plan time between workouts for your body to relax and heal.

Put it on paper. A written strategy may motivate you to remain on track.

3. Get started

Now you're ready for action. As you begin your fitness program, keep these tips in mind:

Start softly and build up progressively. Give yourself plenty of time to warm up and cool down with moderate walking or light stretching. Then speed up to a rate you can sustain for five to 10 minutes without feeling unduly exhausted. As your stamina increases, progressively increase the amount of time you exercise. Work your way up to 30 to 60 minutes of activity most days of the week.

Break things up if you have to. You don't have to complete all your exercise at one time, so you may weave in movement throughout your day. Shorter but more-frequent workouts produce aerobic advantages, too. Exercising in small periods a few times a day may fit into your schedule better than a single 30-minute session. Any quantity of exercise is better than none at all.

Be inventive. Maybe your training program comprises several activities, such as walking. But don't stop there. Find activities you love to add to your workout program.
Listen to your body. If you experience discomfort, shortness of breath, dizziness, or nausea, take a rest. You may be pushing yourself too hard.
Be adaptable. If you're not feeling well, permit yourself to take a day or two off.

4. Monitor your progress
Retake your fitness assessment six weeks after you start your program and then again every few months. You may realize that you

need to increase the amount of time you work out to continue developing. Or you may be pleasantly delighted to discover that you're exercising exactly the appropriate amount to fulfill your fitness objectives.

If you lose motivation, create new objectives or attempt a different hobby. Exercising with a buddy or attending a class at a fitness club may help, too.

Starting a fitness regimen is a crucial choice. But it doesn't have to be an overpowering one. By preparing properly and pacing yourself, you may build a healthy habit that lasts a lifetime.

Chapter 3

Nutrition

Nutrition principles that will power your exercise
What you eat, and when, has a huge influence on your energy level and how well you recover after an exercise.

Rule 1: Pay attention
You may be shocked how many busy individuals underestimate the significance of dietary fundamentals – and then run short on vital nutrients.

Not receiving enough vitamins, minerals and other nutrients might impair your health and your performance.

Yet fuelling up for action is as simple as following the well-established guidelines of a balanced diet: Eat lots of fruits and vegetables, ingest lean proteins, eat healthy fats, get your whole-grain carbs, and drink plenty of fluids, particularly water.

Rule 2: Fuel up (even if your objective is to lose weight) (even if your goal is to lose weight)
Give your body the energy it needs to accomplish the task you desire – even if you are attempting to lose weight.

Skimping on nutrition may diminish muscle mass, weaken bone density and create tiredness. This puts you in danger of injury and sickness, increases recovery time, causes hormone disorders, and, for women, menstruation complications.

Make sure your food plan delivers enough nutrient-dense calories so you can exercise and remain injury-free and healthy.

Rule 3: Love carbohydrates (you need them) (you need them)

Carbohydrates receive a poor reputation among certain individuals. But research over the last 50 years has demonstrated that carbohydrates aid your body during extended and high-intensity exercise. In fact, the more active you are, the more carbohydrates you require.

But what about the tendency for athletes to consume high-fat, low-carb diets? Evidence reveals these diets don't increase athletic performance and rather harm it at greater levels.

During an exercise, carbs feed your brain and muscles.

Carbs for the ordinary exercise – If you are in decent condition and want to fuel a daily, light-intensity activity, take roughly 3 to 5 grams of carbs for every kilogram of body weight. For someone who weighs 150 pounds (68 kilograms) that's between 200 and 340 grams a day.

Carbohydrates for longer exercises - If you exercise more than an hour a day, you may require 6 to 10 grams of carbs per kilogram of body weight. For a 150-pound individual, that's 408 to 680 grams a day.
Pick nutritious carbohydrates like brown rice, quinoa, whole-grain bread and pasta, sweet potatoes, fruits, and vegetables.

Rule 4: Rebuild with protein
Protein is vital because it delivers the amino acids your body needs to create and repair muscle.

Most research shows physically active persons should consume 1.2 to 2 grams of protein per kilogram of body weight. That implies a 150-pound individual should consume 82 to 136 grams per day. People who aren't active should consume less protein. Aim for 8 grams per kilogram of body weight each day.

Good sources of protein include chicken (25 grams in 3 ounces) and fish (20 grams in 3 ounces) (20 grams in 3 ounces). Those who choose to skip meat might try soybeans (20 grams per cup) and legumes such as beans, peanuts, and chickpeas (approximately 15 grams per cup) (about 15 grams per cup). Eggs, Greek yogurt, cheese, and tofu are healthy sources, too.

Rule 5: Don't ignore fats
Fat is a perplexing issue for many individuals. But it's vital to a healthy diet. Fat offers energy and helps your body absorb vitamins. Some vitamins (including A, D, E, and K) really require fat to adequately benefit your body.

Be cautious to choose unsaturated fats. Good sources include avocado, olive and canola oils, flaxseed, and nuts.

Rule 6: Know what you need pre-workout

If you work out less than an hour at a time, eating throughout the day should provide you with adequate energy. However, to minimize GI difficulties, you may want to avoid eating soon before your workout.

As a general guideline, eat one to three hours before your exercise, even if you are intending to conduct a continuous, high-intensity activity, like a half marathon.

Rule 7: Remember the post-workout 15
Your body utilizes its stored energy sources throughout an exercise. After you workout, you need to replace those nutrients as quickly as possible.

Research shows that consuming meals rich in protein after your exercise (within 15 minutes), delivers critical amino acids that strengthen and repair muscles. This may also enhance the energy your body puts into the reserve to draw on in the future.

You'll want to refill your carbohydrates and water after your exercise, too. One method is to consume a post-workout smoothie.

Chapter 4

How do you workout?

How to Do a Beginner Workout at Home

You don't have to undertake lengthy or challenging exercises to lose weight or improve your health and fitness.
1. Beginner exercises may deliver actual benefits from the comfort of your own home, and most simple workouts for beginners don't involve costly equipment. There's no excuse not to get started.

If you're ready to reduce weight, enhance your confidence, and raise your energy level, begin with any of these basic exercises. Within only a few days, you should start to see gains in your fitness level. Use these techniques to push yourself, and build on your results over time.

Before You Begin
Before you start working out at home, it's vital to take a few preventative procedures. Always with your healthcare physician before beginning this or any other training regimen.

If you have a health issue, such as an injury, a history of heart disease, high blood pressure, or type 2 diabetes, you should consider exercise adaptations to keep safe throughout your workout.

2. Enlist the aid of friends or family to support you on your road to better health. Telling people about your new exercise regimen might assist you to remain accountable.

Lastly, it's crucial to define a goal for your new home fitness regimen. Write up your SMART objective (a goal that is precise, measurable, achievable, relevant, and time-bound) (a goal that is specific, measurable, attainable, relevant, and time-bound). Post it in a position where you will see it regularly.

3. This will act as a frequent reminder of your commitment.

How to Start a Workout Routine If You're Overweight

Workout Length
When you are first starting started, creating a realistic time goal for exercise is crucial. You don't need to exercise for hours every day to receive health advantages. Just a few minutes each day may make a huge impact on the way you look and feel.

If you haven't exercised in a long time, you may be eager to become healthy. This might lead you to embark on tough exercises. Unfortunately, your body may need to start at a slower speed.

"Do everything you can do to get started,"
How Much Do You Need to Exercise to Lose Weight?
Basic Beginner Home Workout 1.

Walking is one of the finest types of exercise for beginners. However, finding adequate time, together with the perfect area to go for a stroll doesn't always pan out. What if the weather isn't cooperating? Or, what if you need to be home at a specific hour to care for a kid or another loved one? Luckily, basic, ordinary tasks may transform into a workout in no time.

Three common actions that burn energy, increase muscle strength, improve balance, and enhance your flexibility. Try executing numerous repeats within a limited time window. For a fast five-minute exercise, perform these separate activities many times.

Getting in and out of a chair. The basic process of sitting down in a chair and standing up needs you to tighten your belly, steady your hips, and activate your leg muscles. Getting in and out of a chair frequently might be a fantastic starting workout to practice at home. This action simulates a squat, which is a basic bodyweight exercise commonly seen in more advanced gym routines.

Walking up and down the stairs. Stairs may quickly morph into a home training challenge. Going up the stairs improves strength in your upper and lower legs. It's also a terrific exercise for your glutes (the muscles in your buttocks) (the muscles in your backside).

Your heart rate rises while climbing stairs, forcing you to breathe more as you ascend, which provides for fantastic cardio. Going up the stairs might be challenging, but going down the steps demands balance and knee stability. Use the handrail as required, particularly when you are beginning out.

Got up and down from the floor. Do you have a yoga mat or an area of soft carpet where you can sit down on the ground? The basic act of sitting down on the floor and then standing up again needs full-body strength, flexibility, and coordination. Functional motions like these can help you gain the abilities required for more sophisticated activities in a gym or an exercise class.

Once you are acquainted with each of these moves, combine all three into a home circuit workout. Do each task up to five times before moving on to the next. Repeat the series two to five times in a row for a comprehensive exercise that you can accomplish from the comfort of your home.

Beginner Home Workout 2
If you don't have enough time to work out at home, try multitasking while performing housework. You might try utilizing chores and sneak in a few strengthening workouts each day.

Sweeping your porch is a terrific method to work out the muscles in my belly. You may also brush away leaves and tone your core at the same time.

The rotating action required in reaching for the broom and sweeping it over your body stimulates the oblique abdominal muscles along the sides of your stomach. Lifting the broom back to the beginning place increases the rectus abdominis (which flexes the torso) and the transverse abdominis (which keeps your torso stable) (which holds your torso steady).

Many domestic activities may turn into a short exercises. For instance, rising on your toes to dust a high shelf helps strengthen your calves. Adding a lunge exercise to your vacuuming regimen works your hips and thighs.

Chapter 5

Easy home workout

The Best Home Workout Routines:\sLet's go through the 7 Best At-Home Workouts so you can start training immediately

A tip on warming up and cooling down
Home Workout #1: Beginner Bodyweight (Start Here) (Start Here)
Home Workout #2: Advanced Bodyweight
Home Workout #3: The 20-Min Hotel Routine
Home Workout #4: High-Intensity Interval Training
Home Workout #5: Attack of the Angry Birds
Home Workout #6: Train like Batman

Home Workout #7: The Star Wars Workout!

Bonus No-Equipment Workout: The Playground Circuit

Can home exercises develop muscle or aid with weight loss?

How to design your own at-home exercise

Let's hop right in!

No matter which home exercise you chose, you should always begin with a WARM-UP.

Warm-up is extremely necessary, to begin with before any activity. It doesn't have to be much, however, give it around five minutes to keep your muscles working and your heart rate up.

Arm circles are a terrific method to warm up for your at-home exercise.

This will help you complete workouts correctly and help avoid injury. You may run in place, perform air punches and kicks, or some jumping jacks.

Advanced Warm-up Routine:

Jump rope: 2-3 minutes
Jumping jacks: 25 repetitions
Bodyweight squats: 20 reps
Lunges: 5 repetitions of each leg.
Hip extensions: 10 repetitions on each side
Hip rotations: 5 for each leg
Forward leg swings: 10 for each leg
Side leg swings: 10 for each leg
Push-ups: 10-20 reps
Spider-man steps: 10 repetitions
The idea isn't to wear you out, but to keep you warmed-up

That's step one.

Completing your selected at-home exercise would be step two.

The Count declares the number "2"
Below, you'll discover 8 sequences you may follow along with!

Home Workout #1: Beginner

This at-home regimen for the Beginner Workout article, is as follows:

Bodyweight squats: 20 reps
Push-ups: 10 reps
Walking lunges: 10 for each leg
Dumbbell rows (using a gallon milk jug or similar weight): 10 per arm.
Plank: 15 seconds
Jumping Jacks: 30 repetitions
We also put it into a fun infographic featuring superheroes, since that's how we roll:

This infographic will show you the 6 exercises required to complete the Beginner Workout.
The above is termed "circuit training," with the purpose being to run through the exercise routine once, then again, then again.

Home Workout #2: Advanced

If the basic at-home exercise above is too simple for you, continue on to the Advanced Bodyweight Workout.

THE ADVANCED BODYWEIGHT WORKOUT:
One-legged squats – 10 each side [warning: super-difficult, only try if you're in excellent enough condition]
Bodyweight squats: 20 reps
Walking lunges: 20 repetitions (10 each leg) (10 each leg)
Jump step-ups: 20 repetitions (10 each leg) (10 each leg)
Pull-ups: 10 repetitions [or inverted bodyweight rows]
Dips (between bar stools): 10 repetitions
Chin-ups: 10 repetitions [or inverted bodyweight rows with underhand grip]
Push-ups: 10 reps
Plank: 30 seconds

Home Workout #3: The 20-Min room Routine

You may do a 20-min exercise in your room itself! Utilize the furnishings to their greatest extent.

You may work out in your room using the various ways:
ROOM WORKOUT LEVEL 1:\sBodyweight squats: 20 repetitions
Incline push-ups: 15 repetitions (feet on floor, hands on edge of bed or desk) (feet on floor, hands on edge of bed or desk)
One-arm luggage rows: 10 repetitions (each arm, use your suitcase as your weight) (each arm, use your suitcase as your weight)
Reverse crunches: 10 repetitions
ROOM WORKOUT LEVEL 2:\sOverhead Squats: 25 reps
Push-Ups: 20 reps
Inverted Rows utilizing the desk or table in your room: 10 repetitions

Reverse Crunches: 15 repetitions
Set the alarm clock to 15 minutes from now and see how many circuits you can complete!

Home Workout #4: High-Intensity Interval Training
A LEGO Wizard
You don't have to go to the gym to undertake High-Intensity Interval Training. You may conduct a comprehensive routine just in your own house!

Unless you have a huge backyard, jogging at home could be tricky.

But you know what doesn't take a lot of room?

The iconic burpee bodyweight exercise!
Burpees!

To perform a burpee:

Start standing up, then kneel down and kick your legs out.

Do a push-up, pull your legs back in, and burst up into a leap.

Try to accomplish 20 reps, then rest for two minutes.

Repeat till you loathe yourself.

Home Workout #5: Attack of the Angry Birds

Little Cute Birds in a row

The Angry Birds Workout is meant to be done while you have 5 or 10 minutes to kill.

Sort of like playing Angry Birds...

If you have time for Angry Birds, you have time for an at-home exercise.

Here's how The Angry Birds Workout Plan works: it's deceptively basic — simply four main motions.

Bodyweight squats

Push-ups

Pull-ups (or inverted rows) (or inverted rows)
Planks
If you don't have time to go through the complete sequence, no problem!

Depending on how much time you have throughout the day, you may perform your full workout at once, or divide up your training into four distinct sessions throughout the day (with each session being ONE of the exercises) (with each session being ONE of the exercises).

Here's an example day for your No-Equipment Workout:

Wake up, perform 40 jumping jacks to warm up, and then do bodyweight squats.
At lunch, you take your luggage (if you're at work, milk jug if you're at home) and perform inverted rows.
After work, you do another 50 jumping jacks and then perform your push-ups.

After supper, you do your planks while watching TV.

You could even break it up over two days if required, but the aim would be to perform it in the full sequence at once.

The original Angry Birds Workout page discusses in full Levels 1-6, but here's Level 3 for you:

Bodyweight squats: 50 reps
Push-ups: 50 reps
Pull-ups: 10 reps
Planks: 3-minute hold
Once you've done the whole workout, you have my permission to pull out your phone and play the real game!

Home Workout #6: Train like Batman

This exercise is broken into two days for you.

Batman No-Equipment Workout Day 1:

Rolling squat tuck-up jumps: 5 reps
Side-to-side push-ups: 5 reps
Modified headstand push-ups: 5 reps
Jump pull-up with tuck / Pull-up with Tuck-up: 5 reps
Handstands against the wall: 8 seconds:

Batman No-Equipment Workout Day 2:

'180 Degree' jump turns: 5 repetitions
Tuck front lever hold: 8 seconds
Tuck back lever hold: 8 seconds
Low frog hold: 8 seconds
This is a rather advanced exercise already, but if you want to go to the next level, check out the main Batman Bodyweight Workout for advice on how to achieve exactly that.

Home Workout #7: The Star Wars Workout!

Do you have access to a corridor that you can take over for a bit?

Then you can perform our Star Wars Workout!

It's meant to be done in a very tiny area, like your home's hallway...

or an escape pod.

The "Padawan" Level of this exercise is:

30-second knee or feet front plank (3 Sets) (3 Sets)
10 aided squats or squats (3 Sets) (3 Sets)
10 doorway rows (3 Sets) (3 Sets)
A 60-second Farmer-carry (Farmer's Walk) dumbbells (or milk jugs) (2 sets) (2 sets)
March in place for 3 minutes of intervals (6 sets of 20 seconds on, 10 seconds off) (6 sets of 20 seconds on, 10 seconds off)
8 raised or knee push-ups (4 sets) (4 sets)
60-second Doorway Leans (2 sets) (2 sets)

Bonus No-Equipment Workout: The Playground Circuit

Do you have a local playground? Why not work out there? If you have kids, you can do it jointly. Or let them ignore you.

PLAYGROUND WORKOUT LEVEL ONE:
Alternating step-ups: 20 repetitions (10 each leg) (10 each leg)
Elevated push-ups: 10 reps
Swing rows: 10 repetitions
Assisted lunges: 8 repetitions in each leg
Bent leg reverse crunches: 10 reps
PLAYGROUND WORKOUT LEVEL TWO:
Bench jumps: 10 reps
Lower incline push-ups: 10 reps
Body rows: 10 reps
Lunges: 8 repetitions each leg
Straight leg reverse crunches: 10 reps
After you've gone through a whole set three times, go down the slide!

Can doing it out at home help me grow muscle?
Can doing out at home help me lose weight?
The answer to both of these: sure!

Let's attack them one by one.

#1) Can doing out at home help me grow muscle?

You can 100% grow muscle mass at home.

With progressive overload, I would want to make the exercises harder and more demanding, therefore placing more pressure on your muscles.

So to grow muscle with home exercises, concentrate on:

Increasing your repetitions.
Decreasing your rest intervals between workouts.

Performing increasingly challenging variants (knee push-ups to push-ups) (knee push-ups to push-ups).
Increasing your time under stress (by moving slower) (by going slower).
That will assist you to create strength and muscle from your casa.

Next up:

#2) Can doing out at home help me lose weight?

You may entirely train at home for a great weight reduction approach.

Chapter 6

Keeping it up

12 Easy Tips to Help You Stick With Exercise

It's easy to persuade yourself out of exercising. Even when you have the greatest intentions to work out, excuses are so simple to find — "I'm too tired," or "I'm busy," or "The weather is horrible."

The correct mindset and a few tactics may keep your workout regimen on track. Use these techniques to remain in the game:

1. Do it for yourself: Studies reveal that individuals who are "externally driven" — that is, they go to the gym merely to look good at your class reunion — don't continue with it. Those who are "internally driven" — meaning they work out because they enjoy it

— are the ones who stick in it for the long term.

2. Take modest steps: You would never attempt to run 10 miles on day one, right? When you do too much too quickly, you'll wind up hurting, wounded, and frustrated. Take it easy as you get started. Maybe you merely exercise a couple of hours a day your first week. When it gets simple, you may make it tougher.

RECOMMENDED\s3. Hang tough. No one has flawless form on the first day of strength training. Every exercise needs practice. You'll get the hang of it if you keep making an effort.

4. Mix it up: Do several sorts of exercises to keep things fresh and to train different muscle groups. You don't have to change your whole routine every week, but you do want to vary things around a bit.

5. Don't be your own drill sergeant: Half of all individuals who start a new workout regimen drop it within the first year. It typically occurs because they can't keep up the boot-camp pace they've placed on themselves. It's preferable to work within your limitations, and gradually develop stronger.

6. Bring a buddy: When your inner demons urge you to hit the sofa instead of the treadmill, a workout companion can lead you back on the correct path. It's simpler to bail out at the gym than on the buddy who waits for you there. Studies reveal you'll also work out longer when you have a companion along.

7. Show the clock who's boss: Health experts suggest you should strive for at least 150 minutes of activity a week (30 minutes a day, five days a week, for example), adding weight training at least twice a week. Can't find space in your frantic schedule? Take a

closer look. If you work too late. If you can't complete 30 minutes at once, split workout sessions up into 10- or 15-minute spurts.

8. Get accustomed to it: Your exercise should be just as much a habit as brushing your teeth or eating breakfast. When it's part of your habit, you won't even have to think about it. In a few months, exercise may be a regular element in your day.

9. Live in the now: So what if you skipped a week of training and finished down a pint of ice cream over the weekend? Leave the guilt in the past. You have an opportunity to get back into your routine today.

10. Keep it genuine: You're not going to skim off 30 pounds in a week. Aim for something that's reasonable as a starting step. For instance, expand your fitness plan from 2 to 3 days a week, or exercise for 15 extra minutes each day.

11. Track it: Keep a fitness notebook or use an app to document your progress — for example, how much you walk, or lift and the calories you burn.

12. Celebrate! It takes weeks to notice meaningful effects. Even a pound of weight reduction or a pound of muscle growth is sufficient to congratulate yourself. Go out with pals, or pay for a new pair of pants.

Conclusion

Home Workout and Fitness Tips: Exercising without the Gym
Whether you're working at home, traveling, or social distancing, it isn't always easy to go to the gym. But these techniques might help you remain active and healthy despite your circumstances.
Young lady practicing resistance band exercise.

The significance of being active.
When you're trapped at home, traveling with business, on vacation, or quarantined, it isn't always simple to keep to a workout regimen or maintain your health objectives. You may only have restricted access to workout facilities or find it tough to adapt to a new program. Perhaps you miss the companionship of your gym, the familiarity of swimming laps in your neighborhood pool, or the social connection from walking

or hiking with your regular group of exercise pals. If you're accustomed to attending a fitness class with a motivational teacher, you could also be disappointed with the intensity of exercises on your own.

Maintaining an exercise program at home or in a hotel room might feel more like a 'should' than a 'want to. And with so many of us out of work and suffering financially, having a gym membership and remaining active might feel like much less of a priority. However, even a tiny bit of movement may make a tremendous impact on how well you think and feel. In truth, exercise is one of the most effective tools we have for remaining physically and psychologically healthy—and you don't need access to a gym or pricey health club to gain the results.

Exercise may help reduce sadness, stress, and worry, and assist in the treatment of chronic illnesses, such as high blood pressure and diabetes. By finding new methods to get moving and remain motivated, you can take responsibility for your mood and well-being, preserve a feeling of control during these days of tremendous uncertainty, and stay on track with your fitness objectives even when your typical routine is disturbed.

[Read: The Mental Health Benefits of Exercise]

Exercise and your immune system
While being fit won't prevent you from contracting the virus, it does offer numerous additional preventive impacts. Physical exercise produces endorphins, chemicals in your brain that refresh your mind and body, and it may assist to enhance all areas of your health. In addition to increasing your mood and enhancing sleep, exercise may help enhance your immune system.

But don't overdo it. While moderate physical exercise enhances immune function, too much intensive activity—especially if you are not accustomed to it—may have the opposite impact and depress your immune system.

If you utilize exercise to maintain your energy and spirits at hard times such as these, you may be less prone to resort to harmful coping techniques, such as drinking too much, which can also wear down your immune system.

Making a workout plan to keep you motivated

Planning is crucial to starting and sustaining an exercise regimen. When establishing an exercise regimen, consider any continuing health difficulties, the time you have available, and your energy and stress levels. Many individuals report feeling weary recently from all the pandemic-related worry, so if you're still balancing educating your kids and working at home, or are jobless and concerned about money, now may not be the time to attempt a hard new workout routine.

Whatever your circumstances, make sensible objectives centered on things you like. You're more likely to adhere to a fitness routine if you start modest, recognize your victories, and build up gradually.

Prioritize your exercises. People who place their exercise activities on the same schedule as their regular appointments prefer to stick to their plan. You wouldn't cancel your appointment with your dentist because you were busy with work or simply didn't feel like it at that time. Rather, you'd perform your commitment and then return to work later.

Workout at the time that's appropriate for you. Many individuals who continue a long-term fitness routine train in the mornings. Completing your workout program in the morning may revitalize you and establish a great tone for the rest of the day. Others find it useful to take a break from work and get exercise in the afternoon when their energy is dropping. A surge of movement may excite the brain and help you push through the remainder of the chores on your to-do list.

Be explicit in your goals—and monitor your exercises. Rather than attempting to "get in better shape," select a clear objective such as "walk 30 minutes in the morning on Monday/Wednesday/Friday/Saturday." Try one of the numerous fitness monitors or smartphone applications available to maintain a record of your progress—or just use a calendar to write the duration of your exercise, distance, and effort level. Tracking your progress may help keep you responsible, create a feeling of success, and motivate you to keep going.

Say it out loud. Tell a buddy what your objectives and habits are or publish them on social media. You're less likely to skip a session if you know your friends will be asking about how you got on. And if they offer you favorable comments, it will give you a lift for your next session. Working out with a partner may also help keep you on track, even when you can't be physically together. Set up regular times to work out with each other over a phone or video call—and provide each other support and encouragement.

Keep your exercises interesting. Watch your favorite streaming program or listen to a podcast or some amazing music while working out at home or in a hotel room. Or try action video games or "exergames" that resemble dancing, skating, soccer, bowling, or tennis. These may be fantastic alternatives if you're unable to engage in the actual thing.

Create a home exercise space. If you have a room available, choose a pleasant place in your house to exercise and keep your equipment ready. Try utilizing resistance bands, water bottles, or your own body weight to execute resistance workouts. You may start by performing push-ups against the wall then move to do them against the kitchen counter, the coffee table, and lastly the floor. Have stairs in your home? Stair climbing is an effective strength training exercise. Keep one foot on a step and step up and down multiple times (or try stepping up two stairs for an even harder exercise) (or try stepping up two steps for an even tougher workout).

Find engaging group courses online to keep you motivated
It's so much easier to keep up an exercise routine if you're part of a group that will help keep you encouraged and accountable
Build more activity into your day

Many of us are spending more and more time sitting—watching TV, working at the computer, being on Zoom meetings. But even when you're working at home, you can still find ways to include more exercise into your day. Try to conceive of physical exercise as a lifetime option rather than as a scheduled event. Getting up every 30 minutes for a small bout of movement might pile up during the day.

Intersperse domestic duties with your sitting time: vacuum a room, clean a sink, do some yard work, or wipe down your appliances.

Move about while you are on a call, stand for an online meeting, perform squats or lunges while you're waiting for a meeting to start, or jump jacks in front of the TV during the credits or commercial breaks.

Try 'microwave exercises' (brief bursts of activity) like countertop push-ups while you are waiting for the kettle to boil or toast to pop up.

That said, the current suggestion for adults is to strive for at least 150 minutes of moderate-level exercise per week (or 75 minutes of strenuous intensity) with two sessions of strength-building activities each week. That's around 30 minutes of activity, five times each week. Things are also acceptable to break it up. Two 15-minute workouts or three 10-minute exercises might benefit you just as much. Include warm-up and cool-down time as part of your workout—as well as heavy chores around the home or garden.

Reward yourself
When circumstances make it impossible for you to indulge in your favorite types of exercise, it's reasonable to feel a bit disappointed. Don't beat yourself up but keep trying with various routines until you discover something that you like. And if you feel your drive to begin moving start to fail,

think about how much better you'll feel after even a little activity.

It also helps to offer yourself an additional treat as a reward for sticking with a new fitness routine. Take a long, hot bubble bath, for example, prepare a fruit smoothie, or contact a friend or family member. And remember: the good habits you establish today may enable you to remain healthier and happy well.